Contents

Michelle Lally Lmbt, CA, AAT 704-929-9757 www.MichelleLally.com

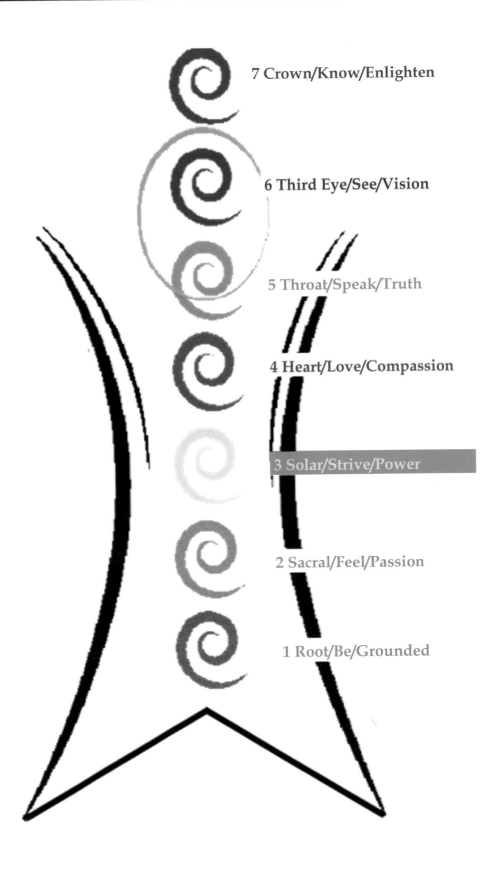

7 Crown/Know/Enlighten

6 Third Eye/See/Vision

5 Throat/Speak/Truth

4 Heart/Love/Compassion

3 Solar/Strive/Power

2 Sacral/Feel/Passion

1 Root/Be/Grounded

Have you ever wondered why we yawn?

Why animals don't move until they stretch? I mean really, really stretch. No matter how much you try to hurry them up, they don't move until they stretch.

Why don't we do that?

I believe we are supposed to stretch and yawn in order to align our entire mind, body and spirit, especially when we cannot control the yawn. It's our body's way of rebalancing.

Did you know that the colors of each chakra are in the same order as the colors of the rainbow? I don't think that is a coincidence, do you? Perhaps a connection between our outer and inner worlds.

After lots of hours of listening to audio books and from what I have witnessed through working with people, I want to share what I have learned. These are just my observations and opinions. I do not in any way claim to medically cure any disease or conditions. I have only listed this information for the purpose of having another tool to assist the body in the healing process.

I feel like I am not here to teach you but to remind you of what you already know. There are thousands of reference books and websites to look up chakra information.

My intention is to offer compiled source for each chakra in relation to body awareness, using breathing and stretching, colors, and essential oils to open up and clear the energy (Nadi) areas that may be blocked. This leaves your joints and muscles surrounding with a refreshed and open feeling.

If you can remember any of this as you go through your day whether it be driving in your car, in the morning before you get out of bed, or in the evening before you sleep, then I will have made a difference in your life by just sharing what I know. Sometimes we just need to be reminded.

So let's get started.

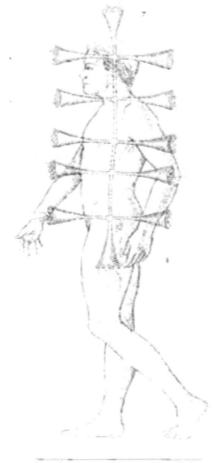

Figure 2-5 Location of the Seven Major Chakra

Chakra's are energy crossroads of life force balance in our bodies. Affected positively and negatively by our beliefs, teachings, limitations, blessings and awareness. Each Chakra can be seen as a pair of cone like vortexes emanating from the front and the back of the body. Together, these vortexes regulate our conscious and unconscious realities, the psychic and sensory energies and our sublets and physical selves. A chakra is a circular-shaped energy body that directs life energy of physical and spiritual well-being. There are many definitions of chakra , but they all evolve from the Sanskrit meaning of the word: "wheel of light". Western tradition frequently attributes the chakra system to the Hindus. The truth is that chakra systems have endured in all corners of the globe. Even before quantum technology of measurement. There have been teachings and knowledge, very precise and accurate . Which always amazes me that this precise knowledge was given to us thousands of years ago for us to be aware of and use for healing. Our cultures throughout the years have untaught us so to speak, our in-

Figure 13

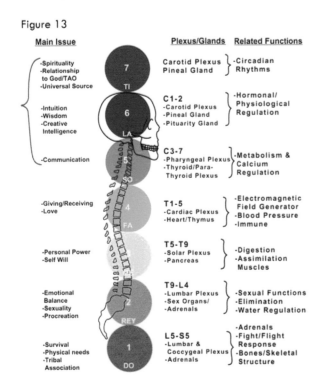

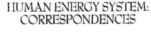

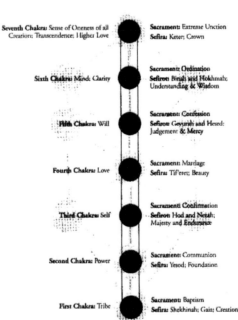

I think of breath as a way to move energy through the body. Of course we know physiologically what each breath does to the blood system as the lungs push oxygen into our blood stream. Well, what happens when we don't breathe? If you think about it, most people go through life not even thinking about their breathing. When we don't breathe all the way filling up our lungs and emptying them each breath, it forces the body to compensate for lack of breath/ oxygen/nutrients/ information. Causing disease (dis/ease) or lack of information/ stress in various parts of our bodies. With lifestyles today, it does not surprise me that most people hold their breath more than they breathe. Let's think about what happens when we hold our breath even if just for a few seconds. Most the time without intention we take a breath in and hold it until the emotion goes away or our thought patterns change.

Observe a baby someday, as long as they are healthy and in homeostasis, they just breath without interruption. Then as life happens we sort of unlearn to breath so to speak, and we can end up with stuck energies in different parts of the body, which play a big role in the chakra balancing flow. So now let's factor in the benefits of Aromatherapy as we breath in the oils and how they enter the body to affect the many different systems. When we use these oils with intentions of specific chakra work the results are extremely enhanced.

I try to at least remember once a day more if I can to take ten deep cleansing breaths/ Prana. With each breath I try to say a positive affirmation, or say something I am grateful for. Adding the essential oils that have the same vibration frequency enhances the experience. In the following pages I have compiled a large amount of information for each chakra to be used as reference. If you need more information on any individual Chakra please Google it and you will be led to the exact page you need for what you need at that perfect time.

When I hear certain sounds or music, it can promote certain feelings, good or bad. When we smell a certain smell it changes the emotional state of being as well. Energy shows up and connects to us in many different ways and it does affect our human body forms to the very deepest cell.

So put on some good music, choose your favorite essential oils, surround yourself with your favorite colors and think positive healthy thoughts. Enjoy the rest of this information.

There are seven main energy centers that vibrate at different frequencies to move energy throughout the body system. These frequencies can be disrupted or blocked by all sorts of energy shifts. Stress or trauma of any kind can alter the flow of energies. As I work my way up the body. I can often feel energy stuck in different parts of the body. I like to start in the first chakra at the feet. Opening and allowing the energy to flow freely while I work up the bodies energy flow regions.

If we use the map of the body from the ground up on our path to self—discovery, we explore our history and planetary roots:

(the feet and the legs); basic survival needs

(the anus and first chakra region); sexual drives and primary interpersonal relationship

(the genitals and the second chakra region); raw emotion, power drives, and social identification

(the belly, the lower back, and the third chakra region); compassion, love, and self-expression

(the chest, the arms, the upper back, and the fourth chakra region); thought, communication and self-identification

(the throat, the neck, the jaw, and the fifth chakra region); expanded mental powers and heightened self-awareness.

(the face and the sixth chakra region); and on toward self-realization or enlightenment (the seventh chakra region)

Ideally when working it is best to unblock each chakra region in order of ascension, but it most definitely is not required. Those who leave unresolved tension in the lower chakras run the risk of contaminating the more sensitive concerns and elements of the upper chakras. I have found that as you do the chakra work it can unravel like an onion. So if you have done the work on the first chakra on one day, ten days later when working on the fourth chakra you may find you need to go back and do some more first chakra work. This work can bring up feelings or emotions that you have not remembered in a long time. Some come to us right away and others may not show up till hours, days or even months later.

The best way to heal any emotional release is to do forgiveness/gratitude work around the negative and the positive thought pattern that come up while working with chakras. I like to check the area either with a pendulum or just use my senses while checking in with the client or myself. Working through these areas starting at the toes/feet and working your way up the body, slowly, talking or thinking about each chakra, can release a lot of emotions. It is important not to judge or criticize but to pay attention to what opens up and then breathe or have them client remember to breath with intentions to release it, replacing it with good energy. It is important we learn to accept ourselves and love ourselves unconditionally and without judgment.

By acknowledging thoughts, feelings, or emotions and turning them into loving positive thoughts of gratitude and forgiveness, we can release the negative energy stuck in the body. By learning about each chakra as much as you can and using some of the knowledge to connect to the energy, is the best way to open up the flow of energy for negativity to be released and most important, open it up so that positive can also flow into the areas. By first learning about ourselves and our emotions, then learning to understand and love ourselves first in relation to each chakra region, we can then allow others to understand and love us and we are ready to face the world and those very same stresses no longer bother you. If you can get your thoughts, feelings and body to the feeling of openness and peace, try to remember what that feels like. That way when your off balance or energy is not flowing you will be able to identify it. When you're out of balance, you will feel off or out of sorts or it will show up somewhere in your physical body system to remind you. You may find that things or situations irritate you more than they have before. The feeling of being in balance or openness may only last a few moments at first but the more you do this and remember the feeling, the deeper the healing can take place and the longer you will feel at peace/balance. There is no right or wrong way to do it. As long as the intention is done with love, light, forgiveness and gratitude, only good can come from it. Enjoy your journey through each chakra.

First Chakra

Physical survival Power Center

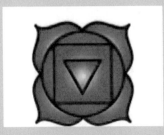

Muladhara/ Base/ Root

Physical survival power center

All my needs are always met

The universe supports me in all that I do

The universe will not let me fall

My unseen friends are always helping me

I am not alone

I am safe and secure

I am my own security

Everything I need appears effortlessly

I am abundance

I feel confidence

The first chakra is the connection to our families or tribe, this chakra can hold energy in it good and bad generally from our beliefs that we are taught by the families we are born into, choose to marry into and choose to raise. The first chakra shares the same energy as baptism or tribal acceptance. It is connected to creation. This is the family we chose to be with to learn the lessons we need in this lifetime. I find that a lot of people hold energy in these areas and symptoms will show up that vary from feet problems to hip problems. It is important to do a lot of forgiveness and gratitude work in this chakra related to immediate or distant/ extended family issues. Whatever we perceive our family issues are in our lives, they are here for us to learn from. To forgive or be grateful not only those who have wronged us, but also for that/those we have wronged. Once the lessons are learned and forgiveness has been achieved, we can feel at peace, open and confident in and around the first chakra areas. Lots of people live their whole lives blaming their parents for the well being good or bad. In previous generations people never spoke of harm done to them by their family members. It was an unspoken secret. It the 60s and 70s that changed and we were taught to speak up and speak our minds. Sometimes too much freedom of speech for then we became victims and we lived as victims . Now things are shifting. Since back in the late 70's and 80 we are learning/ remembering differently. Some of the information I found was written 500 or more years ago. Information my parents had no clue about. Information I will definitely be sharing with my kids and the future generations. Imagine what kind of shift we can make to do the work in this chakra and be able to pass along the new healing memories of peace and gratitude. Of do onto others as you would have done on to you.

Location: Base of the spine,

Energy effected by or effecting: L5-S5 vertebrae, survival, physical Needs, tribal association. lumbar & Coccygeal Plexus, Adrenals, Fight/Flight response, bones, skeletal/structure, Smell, attraction, security, survival. Procreation, food, shelter, safety, feet, legs, ovaries, testes, kidney, bladder, excretory functions, skin, skeletal and muscular systems, cancer, fluid retention, sciatica, patience, grounding, relating, letting go. Accident prone, dependant personality, identity crisis, week ego structure, hoarding, chronic fatigue, predatory behavior, abandonment issues, eating, obesity.

Color vibration: Red, Element: Sound: C, Oohm /Do

Infrastructures of chakra cone:

Back: Unconscious security issues: How others security issues affect you.

Front: Interface with everyday life; How you carry yourself in your world.

Inner Sphere: Is regulated by your souls relationship with the divine

Outer Sphere: Your movement in the world. Over functioning causes jarred and hyperactive behavior. Under functioning creates sloth and laziness

Religious: Baptism, Tribe, Shekhinah; Gaia;

Essential Oils :

Angelica Root Angelica Archagelica/root/base: feeling blocked or cut off from their higher self, guides or higher information, survival, living on the planet and grounding, support, high anxiety, fear, depression and instability, help release negative feelings from traumatic events, revitalization and restoration, feelings of hopelessness, fatigue and stress related disorders

Cedarwood: Cedrs Atlantica/Wood/Base note: Grounding Calming, Strength, great for times of chaos or conflict and meditation

Patchouli: Pogotemon Cablin/Leaves/Base note: Calming, Grounding, aphrodisiac,

Vetiver: Vetiveria Zizanoides/Roots/Base note: Soothing, calming, destress, anxiety, anger, burnout/exhoustion, fear, insecurity

Healthy well-grounded feet and the way a person uses them for support and balance are excellent indicators of how stable and grounded a person is physically and emotionally.

Flat Feet—indicate ungrounded, "hockey puck" way of relating to the world, tends to slide along the surface of the planet. Never putting down roots, never standing still, difficult time staying still in relation to other people and responsibilities.

Clutching Feet—unnatural clutching stance tends to distort the muscles in the feet, locking issues into the muscles tissue. Has a clenched attitude, wants to run away has over developed thighs, need for self control.

Ankles and Knees— act as crossroads, mediate between the forces, physical and psychological, that flow through them.

Weak underdeveloped legs—difficulty grounding himself, hard to stand on own two feet, tentative self image, dependant on others for support and confidence. Massive, over muscled legs— reflect rigid personality, spends great deal of time holding on, difficult time with change.

Fat, Underdeveloped legs— extremely sluggish, difficulty initiating action, following through, on energetic activity, congested way of being in the world, weighed down, unable to lift himself up and outward into life. Thin tight legs—go-getters, intense vital, flow in fits and spurts, points of conflict and dis-ease in joints. Need to mobilize himself through the world, lack of ease and fluidity, not consistent.

Other areas that can be affected by the stress and how our muscles shape our bodies can be the buttock and anal region. Some of the observations are: pinching in of buttock, tight ass, holding on to all his expressions and feelings; pulling in and up of pelvic floor and hamstrings, controlling ones position in life, restricts sexual function, difficulty giving and taking. Holding from the higher muscles in the back and internally, suppresses emotions, overemphasized intellectual control, blocked feelings, digestive disorders

Second Chakra

Creativity & Sexuality Power Center

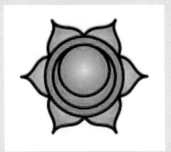

Svadhisthana/ Sweetness/ Below Naval

I am creative

I have great ideas

I posses unique talents

I am confident in my abilities

I am sexy

I have a healthy sexual appetite

I love my body

I love my sexuality

I chose this gender to learn my lesson and

Fulfill my purpose in this lifetime

The second chakra is our connection to our community. It shares the same energy as communion or Yesod. It is the foundation of our belief in who we are in relation to our community. It initiates the expansion of one's individuality, emotional relationship to others, what others think of or what we think of others. It can be financial , spiritual, or self belief. The issues that show up in this area can range from lower back pain, a rash on our waist, to ovary and prostate issues. Stress is held in this area that can range from money to the ability to create life. The beliefs are directly related to what we have learned and how we have processed our first chakra issues. Our belief in ourselves in relation to what we were taught by our families in relation to our sexual identity. You can't do this because you're a girl. Or you're a man you have to be this way in life. It is very important that we work on these issues in our second chakra and do the forgiveness/gratitude work so that we may believe in our self and connect with our community in a positive confident way. I believe we have recreated our second chakra as a collective community through cell phones and internet. We have found a way to connect to our soul siblings. And if you are out of balance you can become very attached to who you are in regard to your connection to your community. Balance is key here in order to be able to move forward to ascension and live in a positive healthy way. The second chakra is also our belief in who we are in regards to financial issues. In our community, it has become very important and in many ways, out of balance in our belief that we are a better person because we have more. Or that they are better because they make more money. I think that belief in today's world has been shifted and is slowly becoming less important. We are finding ways to be balanced more as people become aware of their inner potential and not having to rely on money, cell phones, or others opinions in order to become a better positive healthy person. When open and unblocked, you are not overly obsessed with controlling yourself and everyone around you. Use personal power in a way to heighten your own experience and ambitions without hurting others. Appreciate the importance of your feelings and respects those of others. Not only is sexuality and pleasure associated with this chakra, but also nurturing. Here is our desire for nurturing, nourishment, warmth and touch. Denying these desires causes serious imbalances in life. Overindulgences also will cause imbalances.

Location: Lower Abdomen, Below Navel

Energy effected by or effecting: , L4-T9 vertebrae, sacral nerve plexus, bladder, prostate, womb, kidneys, pancreas, spleen, emotional balance, lumbar plexus, adrenals, sexual functions, elimination, water regulation. Taste, tears, emotions, sexuality, desire, pleasure, creation and procreation, socialization, digestion, kidneys, urinary tract, menstrual pain, loss of appetite, power, money, sex, control, fear, passion, self esteem, incest, creativity, compassion, balance of male and female energies, anemia, allergies

Color: Orange Sound Oooh (like in you) /Rey

Religious: Communion, Yesod: Foundation, Svadhisthana which means sweetness.

Infrastructures of chakra cone:

Back: Feelings you unconsciously carry; your unconscious response to the feeling of those around you; Decisions about which feeling of other you will pick up and hold on to and which you will not. Front:: How you express your feelings into the world; Your ability to translate your feelings into creative responses. Inner Sphere: If you disregard the spirituality of feelings, you will be judgmental and unsympathetic to others. If you fail to translate messages behind the feelings, you will be emotional, hypersensitive and codependent. Outer Sphere: Establishes the way you act as a feeling person in the world. Repressed feelings will attract people who exhibit these feelings to you or cause illness. If you hold feelings that are not yours, you will feel crazy and out of control.

Essential OIls:

Bergamot: Citrus Bergamia/peel/top: depression, anxiety, loss of appetite, stress
Cardamon: Elttaria Cardamomum/seeds/middle, uplifting, energizing, stress, fatigue, depression, despair, aphrodisiac
Neroli: Citrus Aurantium/blossoms/ middle: depression, fridgidity, insomnia
Rose: Rosa Damascena/stem/middle: grief, PTSD, insomnia aphrodisiac
Sandalwood: Satalum Album/wood/ base: grounding, calming, inner peace, stress, depression, low self esteem aphrodisiac

Pelvis tipped upward– flat lower back, less sexual energy focus, holds on to sexual feelings, inability to stay focused or grounded in any emotional activity. Feelings are constricted and constrained.

Pelvis tipped downward— extreme curvature of lower spine, tends to be extreme heightening of sexual energy and sexual focus. Very sensual and feeling oriented, strong need for security, rigid diaphragm, withheld anger, tense or weak chest.

Genital Region: Health and vitality in this area will reflect healthy sexual functioning and relating.

Mostly what I found about the physical stress in this area is that the muscle cells hold onto emotional tension and can therefore, cause your body to change it posture to make up for the tension in the muscles that have tighten or become blocked. That causes the internal muscles to adjust and move so they can function. Sometimes causing stress to the surrounding area/ regions including/ sexual organs.

Not only is sexuality and pleasure associated with this chakra, but also nurturing. Here is our desire for nurturing, nourishment, warmth and touch. Denying these desires causes serious imbalances in life. Overindulgences also will cause imbalances.

Third Chakra

Will Power Center

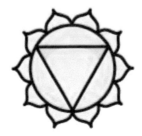

Manipura / Above Naval/ Solar Plexus

I am a strong person

I believe in myself

I can accomplish all that I choose to achieve

I have goals and I will reach my goals

The universe supports me in my entire endeavor

I always work the highest good of all

My will is strong and grows stronger everyday

Thank you Devine creator for such strength and determination

I shall succeed

I am success

I enjoy the beauty of my strong will power

Thank you universe for my growing self confidence

The third chakra is our belief in who we are and how we express ourselves. It can be compared to Confirmation/ Hod/ and Nezah, majesty and endurance. We are confirming who we are in relation to what our families have taught us and who we have become in our community. This area affects our digestive system in relation to how we digest and assimilate everything including thoughts. This center determines the health of our bodies and our minds. Our center for personal power stems from the beliefs we have chosen to learn in relation to the first and second chakras. Stress can show up regarding our power over others or the power we give to others. In this chakra we find balance and decide how we are going to achieve our life purpose, rather than just live out our karma, or past experiences. It affects our motivation, direction, and achievement. By confronting issues of pride and control, you are able to embrace the best features and hold your head high in achievement. The solar plexus chakra has to do with "belonging." If it's open, the individual will feel that he/she belongs to everything--firmly grounded in his/her place within the universe. It's a mental chakra, but directly related to a person's emotional life. Mental understanding of emotions regulates one's emotional life. If the chakra is open, one will have a deeply fulfilling emotional life that does not overwhelm. Also, that person might be susceptible to psychic "attack" or be lost in stars. Physical pain in the chakra stems from overuse. If the chakra is closed, feelings will be blocked. A person might not feel anything and would not understand the deeper meanings of emotions, and might not be connected to his/her greater purpose. This chakra embraces the planes of karma and dharma (ones purpose). Its focus to atone for one's past errors.

.

Location: Above Navel

Energy effected by or effecting: T5-T9 vertebrae, Central or solar plexus, digestive organs and system; muscles and immune and nervous system, pancreas, digestion, assimilation muscles, enzymatic functions, personal power, self will, life force, emotions, pleasure, mental capacity, ambition, arthritis, cancer, coordination, liver, premature aging, stomach, addictive personality, compulsive behavior, excessive anger or fear, manic depression, obsessive, sleep problems, temperamental, driven, need to be recognized and to succeed.

Color Yellow, Sound: Lam Oh (as in go) /Me

Religious: Confirmation, Hod and Nezah: Majesty and Endurance

Infrastructures of chakra cone:

Back: Your unconscious beliefs about power, success, and your deserving of both. Front: Your ability to succeed in the world. Inner: Frequency is established by your internalized beliefs about your place in the world. Do you believe the divine has special work for you and that you have unique gifts? If you do, you will feel healthy and balanced. If you do not, you will feel strained and continually disappointed in yourself. Outer: Maintains your boundaries with the world. If you believe your work is divinely guided, you will perform well and command respect.

Essential OIls:

Ginger Zingiber officnale made from the roots middle base note: uplifting, grattitude, motion sickeness, instability

Juniper Berry: Juniperus communis/ Berrie/ Middle: cleanse, purify, eliminate false or negative feelings, calming, ease stress

Grapefuit: Citrus Paradisi made from the peel top note: letting go, confidence, happiness, peace, contentment

Cypress: Cupressus sempervirens made from branches leaves middle note: uplifting, strength, comfort

This region manages the digestive process and organs, also influences the nervous and immune process. Emanates from the navel and connects with the spine at the eight thoracic vertebra.

When open and unblocked you are not overly obsessed with controlling himself and everyone around. Appreciates the importance of his feelings and respects those of others. Uses personal power as a way to heighten his own experience with out crushing others with ambitions.

When blocked, might lose control if his own emotions, if directed inward might overwhelm with intensity, or if directed outward might encourage to conquer everyone and everything around him, forcing all to conform to his way of thought.

The Belly: Feeling center of the body mind, emotions and passions originate. Where we give birth to feelings, emotions seem to grow out of our guts. Emotions are "energy in motion" (e-motion). Emotions can flow downward, surging through the pelvis and legs.

Acts as the mediator between top and bottom halves of the body mind.

Lower Back: Abdominal stress and tension are frequently at the root of lower back pain. The degree to which a person holds tension in his lower back indicates how compulsive or impulsive his is in his day-to-day activities and relationships. Tension in these muscles reflect the degree of individual over structures and over controls in life.

Diaphragm: Muscle that rests below the lungs and just above the stomach, solar plexus, pancreas, liver, gall bladder, duodenum, and kidneys. Its health and vitality are crucial to the full functioning of internal organs and lungs. Gateway through which the feelings generated in the lower three chakras pass as they ove to the upper portions of the body mind. When open: unblocked, energy flows freely and the body mind experiences health and pleasure. When tight or restricted, result is a limitation of feelings, breathing potential, and energetic flow. Personal defense against unwanted feelings. Stifles emotions. Severe armoring can mean withholding severe and potentially violent rage. Lordosis, nervous stomach disorders, nausea, ulcers, gall bladder, liver conditions.

Fourth Chakra

Love and Compassion Power Center

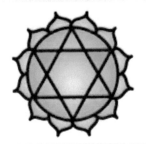

Anahata / Hesod/ Beauty

I am love silently knowing myself

I accept my soul siblings as they are

Knowing we are all there to learn to love ourselves

I see the light with in others

I see the light with in myself

I am worthy of love

We are all worthy of love

I release the need to judge

I release the need to learn from pain

I choose to learn my lessons from love and joy from now on

Thank you universe for all the love you are constantly sending me

I feel the love

The fourth chakra carries the same energy as Union / Marriage / Love. Not just the love of someone else but the love that we have inside for ourselves. The way that we love ourselves, directly impacts our health. The heart itself, has been proven to contain same type of memory cells that are found in the brain and also in other major organs of the body. What is most important to me is that we learn and believe that the love we have for ourselves is the same as what we want to attract. Not only from a lover, but also from all our external and internal relationships including our relationship with spirit, the way we were taught to love ourselves from our parents, our community or tribe. Most of us have never even thought about it. How are you loving yourself so that you children can learn the same behavior? Do you love and take care of your feet? When was the last time you loved your butt? So as we work on the lower three chakra issues we want to keep in mind where we want to be with ourselves in our heart, so that we can ascend to the higher chakra levels. Have you heard the saying green with envy or jealousy? I believe that comes from a insecurity in ourselves and that trust, jealousy and envy all are created in our lack of love and belief in who we are. Doing forgiveness / gratitude work around the feelings of love, weather it being loving to much or not enough, will definitely open up some big issues to work with. Take a deep breath, fill up your thoughts and body with the color green and the feeling of love. See what comes up for you.

"The love (at the fourth chakra) we feel is felt toward everything we encounter, because it is felt within as a state of being. At the heart, our love is no longer one of needs or desires........Love at the heart chakra is one of joyous acceptance of our place among all things, of a deep peace that comes from lack of need and of a radiating quality that comes from harmony within the self."

Location: Center of Chest

Color: Green Sound:: Yam, Ah/Fa

Energy effected by or effecting: Thymus, heart, Lungs, respiratory, cardiovascular, lymphatic, immune, circulatory, heart, high blood pressure, lung cancer, upper back problems, arms, and hands, love of others, compassion, harmony, existential fulfillment, at war with yourself, feelings of alienation, inability to bond with another, self destructive tendency, devotion, compassion, selfishness. Hope, anxiety, endeavor, possessiveness, arrogance, incompetence, discrimination, egoism, lustfulness, fraudulence, indecision and repentance

Religious: Union, Hesod– Love, Sifira, Tiferet; Beauty

Infrastructures of chakra cone: The Chest: primary feeling focuser, amplifier, and translator. Processes emotions, thoughts, reactions, and expressions changing form and direction from creation to expression.

Essntial Oils:

Bergamot: Citrus Bergamia made from the peel. Top: depression, anxiety, loss of appetite, stress

Chamomile: Anthemis nobilis made from the flower middle note: psychological problems, calming, pms, antidepressant, sedative

Cypress: Cupressus sempervirens, made from branches leaves middle note: uplifting, strength, comfort

Marjoram: Organum majorana made from leaves, middle note: opens up, calming, gets energy moving, soothing

The thoracic region extends from the diaphragm upward to the clavicles and consists of the rib cage and its contents, the upper back, and the arms and hands.

The Chest: primary feeling focuser, amplifier, and translator. Processes emotions, thoughts, reactions, and expressions changing form and direction from creation to expression.

Narrow underdeveloped chest, fragile chest: Emotional weakness, insecurity, and depression.

Large overdeveloped chest: Overprotecting of self, losing contact with the more tender aspect of self, feeling tough, strong, blocking gut feelings, don't bother me attitude.

The lungs: primary function is to regulate inhalation and exhalation of life— supporting air/ prana/ life force. Through out the body. Most of us use a small percentage of our breathing potential, using only a small portion of life force that is readily available, affecting overall energy levels.

The Heart and seventh cervical vertebrae: Primary function is experience and expression of affection and love as well as expressive actions generated by feelings. Tension can mean over self-protection.

Shoulders, arms, hands and upper back: Primarily involved with the doing and expressing, show the way a person handles himself. Well developed or narrow and underdeveloped, tight, rigid, difference in right or left shoulder, forward or backward, bowed rounded, raised, square, forward hunched, harbor emotions such as happy, afraid, angry, sad, tired, depressed, exuberant, overburdened, proud, egomaniacal, and humble.

Arms and hands: channels through which a great many of emotions are expressed: Hitting, stroking, striking, grasping, holding, taking, giving, reaching out, manipulating, feeling, self protecting, self extending. Weak underdeveloped arms, massive over muscled, thin tight, fat underdeveloped,

Fifth Chakra

Communication Power Center

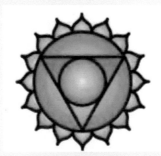

Visuddha /Purification /Confession

I express myself with love

I express myself with confidence

I deserve to be heard

Others are interested in my opinions

I listen to my soul siblings

And they listen to me with compassion

I release the need to be right

I release the need to gossip

I express myself with kindness and compassion

I understand that we all have our own truth

My truth is not the only truth

Thank you universe for the courage to speak up for others and myself

I use the my words for the highest good of all with honestly and integrity

It is in the fifth chakra that we hold energy of Confession. Not just confession of our sins but also confessing our truth. The truth in who we believe we are comes from who we have created our self to be in our lower four chakras. The issues that we have dealt with in life, made us who we are today. This is where we decided how we want to be in our life outwardly. Communicating to others and the words we use reflect what we attract into our energy field. If you speak nice you can usually shift any situation to a nicer more positive vibration. The key is to believe in yourself in any situation to find a positive light to any communication. Are you holding your voice when you should not? Are you speaking too much when you should just listen? The key here is balance. Imbalance can certainly happen in domestic relationships, but it good to be aware that you are speaking your truth an all relationships; work, kids, parents, gym, school, friends etc... It is about giving voice—or music– or sound to our inner heart, and in turn hearing what the world has to reply. This is the last of the chakras that processes the physical elements. Within its location, we prepare to ascend the ladder of consciousness, to shift into the chakras devoted to spirituality. When dealing with issues in this chakra ask what needs to be said to make the transcendence possible. The fifth chakra opens us to higher wisdom, higher guidance, and to our own souls. It is the center of our dreams, if we can determine what truths we really want to represent, we can reach our inner dreams and achieve meaningful lives.

Location: Center of Throat

Color: Blue Sound: Ham/So

Energy effected by or effecting: C3-C7 vertebrae, Pharyngeal nerve plexus, Thyroid/Parathyroid plexus, vocal cords, mouth, ears, vocal communications, expressive; too much or too little, ear, hearing, neck and shoulders, parathyroid speech teeth, throat, self image, self love, self expression, nonstop verbal chatter, poor auditory memory, stuttering, sore throat, stiff neck, colds, thyroid problems, hearing problems, metabolism and calcium regulation

Religion: Confession, Gevura, Hesed, Judgement and Mercy Infrastructures of chakra cone:

Back: The type of guidance you are willing to receive, which can be from lower or higher planes. Front: Determines whish tapes or messages regulate your communication—those that are healthy or those that are not. Inner: What you are willing or unwilling to say or express. How others will perceive your communication. If the frequency is too fast, you are not listening to the divine. If it is too slow, you are listening to lower-ordered beings. Outer: Responds to your intention.

The fifth chakra is the oral segment: Throat, chin, and jaw; Emotional memories and activities correspond to tension and movement in the oral segment of the face. This region is responsible for a wide variety of expressive actions such as talking, crying, laughing, biting, smiling, frowning, smelling, eating, spitting, screaming and swallowing. Health and vitality in this region can be seen to correspond to the uninterrupted flow of such actions and emotions. When these actions are restricted from full animation, blockage and tension may result.

Essential Oils:

Lavender: Lavendula Angutifolia/made form the flower/middle note: Calming, soothing, releases stuck energy in the body, opens energy flow

Eucalyptus: Eucalyptus globulus/made from the leaf/ top note: Opening, freeing, allows movement, stabilizes emotions and concentration.

Geranium: Pelargonium graveolens/made from the leaf/ middle note: antidepressant, opens up flow of life, releases stuck energy.

The fifth chakra is the oral segment: Throat, chin, and jaw

Emotional memories and activities correspond to tension and movement in the oral segment of he face. This region is responsible for a wide variety of expressive actions such as talking, crying, laughing, biting, smiling, frowning, smelling, eating, spitting, screaming and swallowing. Health and vitality in this region can be seen to correspond to the uninterrupted flow of such actions and emotions. When these actions are restricted from full animation, blockage and tension may result.

Tight throat: Fears of expression, breathing is held by the throat., coughing, a tight throat and shallow breathing prevent a true belly laugh, fear of inclusion, soft unintelligible voice .

Bottom of the jaw: Tears are held from prematurely stopped crying, the major jaw muscle (masseter) holds much anger due to inhibitions when young. Masseter tightness determines the position of the jaw, results in overbite, a lisp, violence, any emotion expressed through mouth or face can become fixed in the armor of the throat and jaw, guilt, embarrassment.

Dental problems caused by excessive grinding are often traceable repressed anger.

Receding jaw: Withheld sadness or anger, urge to cry or scream, inability to verbally express any emotion or belief.

Protruding jaw: Defiant character attitude, extremely determined way of being.

Clenched jaw: Over-self control. Swallows or dissolves emotional information.

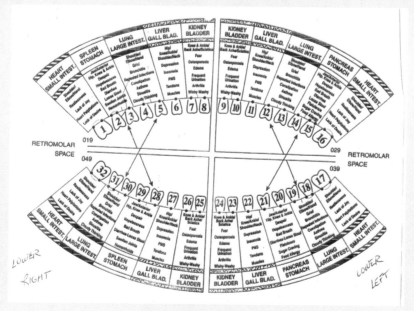

Sixth Chakra

Intuition and Higher Self Power Center

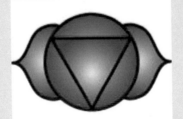

ANJA / To Know / Ordination

I know my higher self communicates with me constantly

I am open to this guidance from my higher self

I listen to my intuition

I release the need to doubt my intuition

I release the need to struggle with decision

I am on my correct path

I know my purpose in life

I accept my spiritual self

I accept my intuitive self

My purpose is for the highest good of all

I trust my higher self

I trust me

Thank you universe for you help and guidance

The sixth chakra has the same energy as Ordination— (the process by which individuals are consecrated, that is, set apart as clergy to perform various religious rights and ceremonies. The process and ceremonies of ordination itself varies by religion and denomination. So this means to me that you really have to know what you believe in for yourself in relation to what you feel from your heart, how you speak your truth and who you believe you are. Once you are in a comfortable place with all of the lower chakra work, you are now ready to just live as if listening and trusting with out a doubt to your intuition or higher power, not ignoring your spirit as it talks through you. You live your life as if you just have an understanding of how things are, what the your purpose in life is and you just be that. Ask yourself; "What do I believe in? Do I live my life in a healthy, positive, giving, loving way? Not just in my outwardly relationships, but also in my relationship with myself and with spirit." As you ask yourself these questions and do the forgiveness and gratitude work, breath in deeply and feel your head open up and your body relax. Put on your favorite music or sit in silence. What ever works for you to just let your thoughts open up. There is no right or wrong. Everyone has their own method of connecting to spirit. And if your not sure what yours is just ask for God/ spirit/ yourself to show you what you need to be able to do this work.

Affirmations to help open and promote healing: I know my higher self communicates with me constantly; I am open to this guidance from my higher self; I listen to my intuition; I release the need to doubt my intuition; I release the need to struggle with decision; I am on my correct path; I know my purpose in life; I accept my spiritual self; I accept my intuitive self; My purpose is for the highest good of all; I trust my higher self; I trust me; Thank you universe for you help and guidance

Location: Center of Forehead/ Third Eye

Color: Indigo Sound: Sham/La

Energy effected by or effecting: C1-C2 Cartotid Plexus, Pineal Gland, Pituitary gland, hormonal/physiological regulation, intuition, wisdom, creative intelligence.

Ears, eyes, forehead, cheekbone, jaw, mouth, knowledge, mind, clarity, meditation, vision, insight, creativity, realization, blindness, headaches, nightmares, eyestrain, blurred vision, brain tumors, Central nervous system, headaches, sinus, extreme confusion, fixations, living in fantasy world, paranoia, poor visual memory, hearing.

Infrastructures of chakra cone:

Related to development of heightened self-awareness. The word 'face' is also used to refer to a person image which relates the concept of face to ego, image a person projects 'to lose face'. To hide your face denotes a sense of shame in which the ego feels humiliated. Strong ego 'faces up' to situations. Weaker ego might 'face away'

Religious: Ordination, Binah and Hohmah; understanding and wisdom

Essential Oils:

Clary Sage: Salvia sclarea/Leaves, tops/ Middle note: Stress, Exhaustion, nervousness, fear, paranoia and depression

Cypress: Cupressus sempervirens/ Branches/Leaves Middle note: uplifting oil can provide strength and comfort, and when inhaled just before bedtime can be soothing and relaxing

Frankincense: Boswellia carteri/ Resin/ Base note: Grounding Calming, Relaxing, great for meditation

Vetiver: Vetiveria zizanoides/ Roots/ Base: soothing and calming. unwind or de-stress. Spiritually, grounding, meditation, prayer, soothing, calming, fear, burn out, exhaustion, insecurity,

Related to development of heightened self-awareness. The word 'face' is also used to refer to a person image which relates the concept of face to ego, image a person projects 'to lose face'. To hide your face denotes a sense of shame in which the ego feels humiliated. Strong ego 'faces up' to situations. Weaker ego might 'face away'

There is the smiling face, depressed face, bright face, sad face etc. Most people are unaware of the expressions on their faces and to that extent are out of touch with who they are and how they feel. Face muscles register tension, and emotions. "I can read it all over your face". Plastic smile, growling, frowning, intellectual, sexy, serious. Etc...

Ears: I can't hear you, good listener, I hear too much, your ability to hear what others have to say. Your emotional state can affect your hearing accompanied by tension in the various neuromuscular regions that surround your ears. Ears contain the semicircular canals that are responsible for maintaining a sense of balance within your body mind, your equilibrium and your feeling of security in the world.

Eyes: Consist of a contraction and immobilization of the greater part of all of the muscles around the eye, eyelids, forehead, rear glands, as well as the deep muscles at the base of the occipital– involving even the brain itself. Eyes are the window to the soul.

Large round eyes: Warm, loving personality, caring attitude.

Bulging eyes: Indicate nervous way of being in the world, reaching out with his eyes, anxious in presence.

Deeply set: Lifetime of withheld expressions, withdrawn sadness, guard and protect, critically observing the actions and activities of others.

Baby eyes: Wide-opened, pleading, doubly expressive, innocent and immature or seductive and manipulative.

Nearsighted: Have difficulty projecting themselves outward, inwardly focused or shy, highly rational and introspective. Can be traced to an early trauma causing him to withdrawal affecting future development.

Farsighted: Inability to perceive activities that are up close, focuses away from self, looks outward, extroverted, outgoing, extends himself in activities and relationships.

Seventh Chakra

Spiritual Power Center

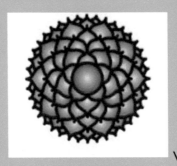

Sahasrara / Understanding / I know

I connect with the universe

I am open to communicate with God

I am ready to become aware of who I really am

I send love and peace out to beings of the universe

I ask for support and guidance from my unseen friend

I work for the highest good of all

I am open to receive love and guidance

I remember who I really am

The seventh chakra shares the same energy as the Sacrament of Extreme Unction or last rights, usually given to those close to death. The last thing before total ascension to heaven or release of your spirit, whatever your belief is about death. I personally think that this is the most important chakra to do work in. You don't have to be dying physically to do your work in this chakra. Death of your old ways of thinking, death of all the things that you have held onto all these years, the death of your old thoughts and replacing them with thoughts of higher power and energy. Death of who you thought you were and forgiveness / gratitude work in and around who you are to become and who you are right now in this very moment. If we get rid of our old thoughts and patterns of thinking, we can come closer to being one with God, knowing we have been forgiven and that we are thankful for all the lessons that have brought us to this place in time on this planet. Keeping this in mind as you work and rework each chakra, will guide us in a direction of ascension. The more we know what our ultimate goal of forgiveness and gratitude is, the faster and easier the road will be in our body, mind and soul. With the discovery and the opening of the 7th chakra, we transcend from the physical to something beyond....a greater consciousness. After all, we are not our bodies, but our minds and souls. We are part of the collective consciousness. We are part of the Great Spirit. Sense of oneness of all creation; transcendence; higher love. The highest extension point for rising energy. Here the "I" dissolves into the greater spirit, creating and opportunity to be ones true self. Someone who lives in this chakra exists in constant revelry of being "self" and "all" simultaneously. Detachment from the physical body and with that, freedom from pains, troubles, and humiliations of the world. But this separation can also lead to impassiveness, aloofness, and a sense of being alone in a group. This person is usually able to manifest through his or her own powers. This presents the amazing opportunity to help others. Many achieve guru status because of their awakened and amplifies gifts. Some individuals confuse being gifted with being special however, becoming egoists. Addicted to the fame or fortune. I would suggest going back and doing more of the lower chakra work to get through this.

Location: Crown / Top of head

Color: Purple Sound : Om , Eee /Ti

Energy effected by or effecting: Carotid Plexus, Pineal Gland, Spirituality, relstionship to God/Tao, connection universe, oneness, cerebral cortex and the central nervous system, depression, alienation, confusion, boredom, apathy, and the inability to learn or compre-hend, baldness, epilepsy, migraine, Parkinson's, excessive gullibility, multiple personalities, nightmares.

Religious: Extreme Unction, Keter

Infrastructures of chakra cone: Back: The types of spirits and spiritual beliefs programming your belief system; sometimes these hold you hostage. Front: How you project your image of the divine and spiritual self into the world; the religion you follow and the values you live. Inner Sphere: If healthy, your spiritual beliefs and discipline will match your purpose and the divines desires for you. If not, there will be discord. Outer Sphere: Reflects how you carry out your spiritual beliefs.

Essential Olls:

Cedarwood: Cedrs Atlantica: Made from the wood, base note: Grounding Calming, Strength, great for times of chaos or conflict and mediation

Frankincense: Boswellia carteri/ Resin/ Base: Grounding Calming, Relaxing, great for medi-tation

Patchouli: Pogostemon cablin/ Leaves/ Middle: Romance, meditation, earthy, grounding,

Neroli: Rutaceae/ Flowers/ Middle::Depression, insomnia, shock, stress, strong emotional support, soothing and calming to the nervous system, trauma, antidepressant, anxiety

The

highest extension point for rising energy. Here the "I" dissolves into the greater spirit, creating and opportunity to be ones true self. Someone who lives in this chakra exists in constant revelry of being "self" and "all" simultaneously. Detachment from the physical body and with that, freedom from pains, troubles, and humiliations of the world. But this separation can also lead to impassiveness, aloofness, and a sense of being alone in a group. This person is usually able to manifest through his or her own powers. This presents the amazing opportunity to help others. Many achieve guru status because of their awakened and amplifies gifts. Some individuals confuse being gifted with being special however, becoming egoists. Addicted to the fame or fortune. I would suggest going back and doing more of the lower chakra work to get through this.

Head/body split: The head and face are our most social aspects. Together they make up the mask we present to the world. We focus more attention on our faces and intellects than on any other place in the body mind. It is considered the resting place for the mind, the intellects and reason. The body on the other hand, is considered to be our emotional, less creative aspect. The split is body/mind, intellect/ feelings, and reason/intuition can all be seen in the way the head and body relate to each other.

Head held forward; usually reflects one who encounters the world first with his head, with his rational self. Races ahead of the body to evaluate conditions before it allow the rest of the body to proceed.

Head tilted to the right: can mean feeling arrogant and defiant, chip on shoulder.

Head tilted to the left: projecting feeling cute and playful attitude.

The bearing of the head is a direct relation to the quality and strength of the ego.

Long graceful necks: reflect long, proud attitude.

Stout, bull necks indicate tight, aggressive approach to life's demands

Earth Element
Essential Oils for Spleen-Stomach Channel
Acupressure Points

This convenient, time-saving way with pure essential oils that activate acupuncture acupressure points along the Spleen and Stomach Meridians. Apply the Earth Element to appropriate acupressure points to initiate physical and emotional balancing. Use this natural self-care remedy with or without pressure on acupuncture points to invoke this ancient healing method. Many of the points along the **Spleen and Stomach Channel address digestive issues**. Apply to acu-points above, below, and at the site of trauma for pain relief that has occurred along the Stomach or Spleen Channels. Contains pure essential oils intended to balance emotions related to the **Earth Element such as worry, overthinking, and lack of empathy.**

Directions for Use: Apply to indicated points 1-3x per day.

10ml Tall Roll-On glass Bottle of Each of the following blends: Ingredients Earth Coconut Oil, Juniper, Tangerine, Spearmint, Fennel and Ginger Essential Oils. -https://agelessherbs.com/

Related Aroma Acupoints:

Acupressure Point Stomach 3

Acupressure Point Stomach 36

Acupressure Point Stomach 37

Acupressure Point Stomach 38

Acupressure Point Stomach 40

Acupressure Point Stomach 44

Acupressure Point Spleen 3

Acupressure Point Spleen 4

Acupressure Point Spleen 6

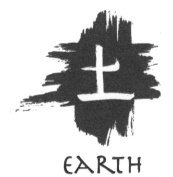

EARTH

For exact location photos on each point or for more specific issues, please fill out my evaluation form, or call/text to set up an appointment.

5 Element Oils Sets Available at MichelleLally.com

Michelle Lally Lmbt, CA, AAT 704-929-9757 www.MichelleLally.com

Fire Element
Essential Oils for Heart-Pericardium Channel
Acupressure Points

This convenient, time-saving way with pure essential oils that activate acupuncture acupressure points on any of the four Meridians associated with the Fire Element. Apply the Fire Element acupressure stick to the related points to initiate emotional and physical healing listed below. Contains pure essential oils that affect emotional balancing associated with the **Fire Element of Chinese medicine such as lack of joy, emotional/sexual coldness, emotional/Shen disorders, and sleep problems**. Has a lovely aroma with high citrus and floral overtones and deep sensual grounding base notes.

Directions for Use: Apply 1-3x per day.

10ml Tall Roll-On glass Bottle of Each of the following blends: Ingredients Fire Coconut Oil, Lavender, Sweet Orange, Frankincense and Rose Essential Oils. https://agelessherbs.com/

Related Aroma Acupoints:

Acupressure Point Heart 7

Acupressure Point Small Intestine 3

Acupressure Point Small Intestine 4

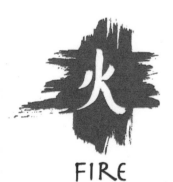

FIRE

For exact location photos on each point or for more specific issues, please fill out my evaluation form, or call/text to set up an appointment.

5 Element Oils Sets Available at MichelleLally.com

Michelle Lally Lmbt, CA, AAT 704-929-9757 www.MichelleLally.com

Metal Element

Essential Oils for Lung-Large Intestine Channel

Acupressure Points

This convenient, time-saving way with pure essential oils that activate acupuncture acupressure points on the Lung Channel and the Large Intestine Meridians listed below. It can be applied with or without pressure for effective self care that initiate emotional and physical balancing. **Many of the points along both Channels help to normalize the respiratory system including the sinuses. Addresses issues** associated with **Metal Element Imbalances including unresolved grief and sadness, lack of spiritual connection or growth, digestive issues, poor personal boundaries, and low self-worth.** This remedy can be used on, above, or below areas of pain or trauma on acupuncture points for pain relief.

Directions for Use: Apply 1-3x per day to indicated acupressure points. 10ml Tall Roll-On glass Bottle of Each of the following blends: Ingredients Metal Coconut Oil, Bergamot, Sweet Orange, Oregano, Cypress and Cinnamon Essential Oils. https://agelessherbs.com/

Related Aroma Acupoints:

Acupressure Point Lung 1

Acupressure Point Lung 7

Acupressure Point Lung 9

Acupressure Point Lung 10

Acupressure Point Large Intestine 4

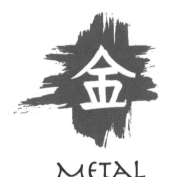

METAL

For exact location photos on each point or for more specific issues, please fill out my evaluation form, or call/text to set up an appointment.

5 Element Oils Sets Available at MichelleLally.com

Michelle Lally Lmbt, CA, AAT 704-929-9757 www.MichelleLally.com

Water Element

Essential Oils for Kidney-Bladder Channel

Acupressure Points

This convenient, time-saving way with pure essential oils that activate acupuncture acupressure points on the Kidney and Bladder Meridians. Apply to acupressure points listed below to initiate emotional and physical balancing. Contains pure essential oils that address psychological issues associated with the **Water Element of Chinese medicine such as lack of willpower, lack of awe, anxiety, and irrational fears leading to panic attacks.** This blend activates acupressure points that assist with issues such as low virility and infertility **as well as other Kidney energetic attributes such as premature aging.** Used along the Bladder channel for back pain and leg pain.

Directions: apply 1-3x per day to indicated points.

10ml Tall Roll-On glass Bottle of Each of the following blends: Ingredients Water Coconut Oil, Lavender, Cinnamon, Eucalyptus, Wintergreen, Sweet Orange, Helicrysum, Clove and Peppermint Essential Oils. https://agelessherbs.com/

Related Aroma Acupoints:

Acupressure Point Kidney 1

Acupressure Point Kidney 3

Acupressure Point Kidney 6

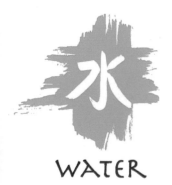

WATER

For exact location photos on each point or for more specific issues, please fill out my evaluation form, or call/text to set up an appointment.

5 Element Oils Sets Available at MichelleLally.com

Michelle Lally Lmbt, CA, AAT 704-929-9757 www.MichelleLally.com

Wood Element

Essential Oils for Liver-Gallbladder

Acupressure Points

This convenient, time-saving way with pure essential oils that activate acupuncture acupressure points on the Liver and Gallbladder Meridians. Apply to the acupressure points to initiate emotional and physical healing. **Pure essential oils work to alleviate emotional constraints leading to depression, anger and frustration as well as physical maladies associated with the Wood Element imbalances according to Chinese medicine such as menstrual disorders and poor sleep patterns.** Use points above, below, and at the site of pain for relief. Acupressure oils are able to activate the points with or without pressure applied

Directions: apply 1-3x per day.

10ml Tall Roll-On glass Bottle of Each of the following blends: Ingredients: Wood Coconut Oil, Lavender, Rosemary, Cedarwood and Lemongrass Essential Oils. https://agelessherbs.com/

Related Aroma Acupoints:

Acupressure Point Liver 2

Acupressure Point Liver 3

Acupressure Point Gallbladder 1

Acupressure Point Gallbladder 14

Acupressure Point Gallbladder 34

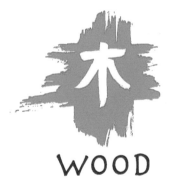

WOOD

For exact location photos on each point or for more specific issues, please fill out my evaluation form, or call/text to set up an appointment.

5 Element Oils Sets Available at MichelleLally.com

Michelle Lally Lmbt, CA, AAT 704-929-9757 www.MichelleLally.com

LIVE AS IF!

What is the one thing I could teach another massage therapist that could improve their practice?
The answer is simple "Live as if."
What does "Live as if" stand for?
It means that we create the life, the business and the customers we dream of having. Live as if your goals are already met. Whether it means that you are the most compassionate massage therapist offering care to those who can't afford it, or most successful with other therapists working for you, or you're the most educated body-worker in your community. Whatever your personal and professional goals are, live as if they have already come true.

We hear people say "I don't have time to get a massage" or "I don't have time to take another class." Yet too often these are health industry professionals who want to attract the kind of person, client or patient that sees the value of self-care. Make a choice to be the person you want to attract to your life, personal or professional. Surround yourself with a community of people who do the same.

For example, I receive a weekly massage, from a therapist who also receives massage, or in other ways takes care of themselves. They believe as I do that it is the most important thing they can do, in addition to other self-care therapies and healthy living regimens. So, I attract customers who also believe in self-care practices.

Ten things to be mindful of

10 swallows of water! Most people put a cup to the mouth and maybe swallow 3 or 4 times, stop and take 10 swallows (of water) each time you put a cup to your lips.

10 Breaths ~breathe in and out ten times don't stop

10 min Stretch as often as you can each day for at least

10 min Meditation that's all it takes, think of something your grateful for, you can compassion for, you feel love for

10 Affirmations~ just ask google/siri/alexa to tell you 10 if you can't think of any.

10 min of walking ~in place counts too, make sure you swing your arms

10 min of smiling ~at yourself in the mirror, your dog, a stranger whatever works...

10 min of feet on the ground (no shoes)

10 acts of kindness (that can mean throwing a love/peace hand sign instead of what you really wanted to

10 min call a friend you have not spoken to, or relative

When I look back on my success as a Bowen Therapy Instructor, Massage Therapist and Retreat Owner, I can attribute it to learning one simple tool:
Live as if!
I have had my own Wellness Center, working with other healthy lifestyle professionals who believe as I do about quality of care for themselves, their family and their community. I attract clients who are seeking a healthy lifestyle and also give back to their community through donations, gift cards or reduced rates for the elderly.

My massage career started at 42, now I'm 60, have two adult children, grandchildren, a loving partner, perfect home/retreat, a successful business and I practice self-care daily. My key to a happy, healthy and abundant lifestyle?
I live as if!

Published in 2018 Massage Magazine

Michelle Lally Lmbt, CA, AAT 704-929-9757 www.MichelleLally.com

SOURCE OF INFORMATION:

Affirmations on each chakra:

YIN Cleansing Meditation With Bonus MANIFESTING!

© 2006 Nuroc Mind Spa & Vicki Webb

The Subtle Body

An Encyclopedia of Your Energetic Anatomy

By Cyndi Dale

Bodymind

By Den Dychtwald

Energy Anatomy

The Science of Personal Power, Spirituality

Caroline Myss, PHD

Various Websites:

http://members.tripod.com/kira_lis/chakra1.html

http://aromaweb.com/essentialoilschakras/chakraessentialoilrecipes.asp

http://www.stillpointaromatics.com/angelica-root-Angelica-archangelicapure-essential-oil

http://www.anniesremedy.com/herb_detail166.php

http://www.auracacia.com/chakras

http://www.paulcheksblog.com/the-body-as-temple

https://agelessherbs.com/

Made in the USA
Columbia, SC
07 May 2024

35337309R00024